Wild for Life

POEMS

MARGOT WIZANSKY

LILY POETRY REVIEW BOOKS

Copyright © 2021 by Margot Wizansky

Published by Lily Poetry Review Books
223 Winter Street
Whitman, MA 02382

https://lilypoetryreview.blog/

ISBN: 978-1-7375043-1-3

All rights reserved. Published in the United States by Lily Poetry Review Books. Library of Congress Control Number: 2021949201

Cover Art: *After the Storm, Mattapoisett Harbor* by Margot Wizansky
Hand lettering: Margot Wizansky
Design: Sasha Wizansky

For David, Ben, and Sasha,
and all the strangers, friends, and family who brought me back

TABLE OF CONTENTS

I Must Have Been Wild for Life / 1
All of it Changes at Evening / 2
Morning Has Come / 3
Last Rites Were Offered / 4
Letting Go / 5
To My Aorta / 6
Where Was August? / 7
Three Months Out, Hoping for Something More / 8
Something Less Than Beauty / 9
Getting It Right / 10
Clarity / 11
Small Talk / 12
Terms of Endearment / 13
Not Bred For Fierceness / 14
Fred Wants to Know if I Believe in God / 15
Temporary Separation / 16
Dignity / 17
My Concerns Are Very Small / 18
Rebirth / 19
Under a Giant Hat / 20
Ode to Your Breath / 21
A Day We Eat Like Gods / 22
After My Year of Being Two-Dimensional / 23
About Their Vigil / 24
Nothing Is the Same / 25
A Meditation on the Present / 26
Tonight Only Poetry Will Serve / 27
Acknowledgments / 29
About the Author / 31

The heart can give out and return
And the scar we share,
The scar is just a line-break.

—VERANDAH PORCHE

I MUST HAVE BEEN WILD FOR LIFE

I held fast to the tiniest bit,
held on down to my very beginning.
Because I felt no agonies, why was I not
joyful, why so quiet and so slow? Joy seizes
the rising moon. Why wasn't I holding
the other end? There's a black line on my chest,
lumpy and scarred. The week of my coma,
what was it, absence or sleep? Memory
does not assail me. It was only my heart
beating. Was I in my body, deep inside,
or had I left? I can't let it in all at once,
just a small portion of blue sky and a yellow
flower whose name I don't know.
Half the garden died while I was recovering
and the other half greets me stiff-armed.
I sit upright and watch the kind of TV
that simply runs my mind. Was I supposed
to have died? Did I? Was I brought back?
I could have slipped over so easily,
the thin margin visible to me now.

ALL OF IT CHANGES AT EVENING

String of cars on the bridge,
    halos from streetlights,
        night-things have their time—
            I don't want the dark in rehab.
    When the big shade draws down,
        semi-opaque, worked with a switch,
I start counting the hours.

At half-past five, the sunlight begins,
    touching the cables,
        the tugboats,
           unless fog closes
the whole landscape, making me
    shut-in and very small.

If it were all right just to love and die,
    I wouldn't be in this place seven stories up.
Thank God for the harbor and the barges
    my husband loves to watch.

MORNING HAS COME

Still gray, but morning enough.
It was a good night. I didn't get hungry,
didn't need roasted nuts, didn't toss
and turn after a trip to the bathroom.
I sip a big mug of foamy hot chocolate
because coffee doesn't suit me these days.
My first memory is moaning. No last.
Completely cared-for, I yielded
everything. My husband pointed out
the USS Constitution in the harbor,
and the dawn touching the Zakim Bridge.
I didn't care about any of it. For weeks,
I didn't see beauty at sunrise,
didn't feel pain, didn't move my body
for hours. I tried to find myself
in my syrupy brain, tried to read,
to write, trying to understand.

LAST RITES WERE OFFERED

My husband buries his head in my neck—
says he wants me back, the old me,
doing five things at once.

He wants to obliterate the details of my collapse
and yet he recites the catalog over and over,
the lonely drive behind the ambulance at 4 AM,

the emergency room offer to call the priest for last rites
he refused. And home now, I do one thing at once,
dress more slowly as the woman I was, put on

one earring, then the other, my pearl necklace.
I ask him to help me with the clasp. I take
a silk scarf from the shelf, comb my hair

in the mirror, examine my scar and below,
the heart monitor attached to my chest.
Maybe he can't see me finishing one task

before I start another, foaming the milk
before I scramble the eggs.
I might always be wary.

LETTING GO

It's the beginning of your letting go.
You've been holding yourself together,
waiting to know I'll survive.

You were most frightened
when you couldn't
communicate with me at all.

Now you're holding me
on your lap in the big chair,
my back to you, and I feel you crying.

I know you're thinking about life
without me, and it will happen,
probably not this time, but it will,

and one of us will have to find a way
to go on. Time was, I had
a limit to being held. I'd push you

away and go on to the next thing.
Today there's only your holding me,
our eyes filling.

TO MY AORTA

You failed me. No warning.
Three layers strong, carrying
blood to every part of me, oxygen
fast riding it like microscopic
submarines, no low tide,
until it tore, and blood surged.
Not through to your outer layer,
the lucky path of the surge
buying time for an army
to pump blood into me to save
my life. I don't know if I can
trust you to tend me.
You're patched with dacron,
whole again. The cardiac surgeon
stitched like a seamstress,
induced a long sleep to give you
room to settle, time enough
for Death to lose interest in me.

WHERE WAS AUGUST?

It wrecked my summer.
My heart opened and took
the hot and sunny days
where August should
have been, sweating
and laughing. Oh, the many
days I have missed,
wondering whether I'll
sleep tonight. Friends think
it should be over. I should
be recovered. Two beds
of impatiens completely
disappeared from my untended
garden, a collection
of spent stems and weeds
and no one looking
after it. I cut the two giant
zinnias that remain.

THREE MONTHS OUT, HOPING FOR SOMETHING MORE

The night, too hot and wet.
Morning comes in the spaces
between the leaves. My head
is foggy, gently tangled, as
those leaves twist and blow.
Today I could cry. Will I get
any better, any stronger?
I'm still awake from 2 to 4 AM
and sometimes longer. My life
is small and it bores me, smaller
than a Kleenex box, it sits
on the end of the sofa.
The spirit leaked out. I want
to be tight with it, as tight
as a tomato in its skin, so tight
I could split. I want everything,
to have poems gush out of me,
to cook dishes I gorge on, to walk
on streets I've never walked, to dig
for giant quahogs that resist
my rake, stay fast in their holes.
An almost sour listlessness
pins me to the chair,
and when I raise myself to stand,
my legs are heavy. I trudge
the neighborhood, knees
shouting. *Stop! Stop!*

SOMETHING LESS THAN BEAUTY

When I finally woke up, I saw they'd taken me
apart and put me back together. I was limp

as a hooked fish and bulging in new places. Nurses
held my arms and I took wobbly steps.

My feet wouldn't go where I wanted them.
I practiced stairs, each one a little mountain.

I was hungry and couldn't eat, the food,
ground up, bland, gray, gritty.

I hoped my leg would lose its numbness
where the tube had been, that my belly

would retreat, and I'd spring up from my chair
like I used to. I wanted sleep, with my mind empty

and expectant, not needing to check the clock at 3 AM.
You carried my magazines, circled me, watched over me,

your presence there asking, *are you all right?*
What can I say when you tell me how much you love me?

GETTING IT RIGHT

I've noticed a groan at the far edge of love.
His compliments pile up like mail unopened.

I have no template for the new me.
Unmoored and drifting, I'm lost

and can't be certain of anything.
I walk into a room, I walk out of a room.

What does it matter? I want reality,
truth that cannot be twisted—

cider flowing from the press, shell collecting,
patching the hole in the screen door.

There are days I see every dirty cigarette butt
on the street, magnified, and days I see colors

too bright, red leaves on the burning bush
that make me turn away. Isn't it hubris to think

our own small unwindowed space is the full
tally of consciousness? No starting over

the great go-round I've got.
I'd better get it right.

CLARITY

Everything takes on an aura
bigger than real and more
luminescent, the sky more clear,
air more crisp, the salvia taller
and more purple. I keep thinking
I wasn't supposed to have
this clarity, wasn't supposed
to be here. I need the confidence
to put one foot on a step
and then the other. When
friends say things unthinkable,
what may once have been
annoying, just passes.
It no longer works, that part
of my brain that leapt to respond.
I just smile and let it go.

SMALL TALK

These mornings I don't speak,
and certainly not of love.

I could be nicer to you
when you want to touch me

with your words, any words,
hold me with a thread of sound.

It's my mother I blame.
Talk frightened her.

She'd scrutinize her nails.
I broke a nail, she'd say,

I have a hangnail, her hands
performing small sad movements,

never still. You only ever wanted
the hum in my throat to answer

the hum in yours. I've been
ruined for the mornings.

TERMS OF ENDEARMENT

Muffin I was when we first got together, soft and top-heavy,
        flesh rolling over my waistband

Muffin going dry and stale in the air, crumbling to the touch

You're Adorable, a huge billboard you've mounted above the highway

Teeny-weeny me, my hand over my eyes so I don't have to see it

Adorable like a kewpie doll with big eyes, and hollow inside

I love you, you say, when there's nothing adorable or soft about me

I love you, you say, when I won't let you take my poem as though
        it were yours, the one that moves you

I love you, you say, when I'm bitching about your old-man noises

I love you, you say, instead of *you're wounding me*

I'm a killer bee. Sorry I can't stop stinging

NOT BRED FOR FIERCENESS

The way it hurtles at me,
trailing its counterweight.

When you want to hold me, I keep
myself a little stiff, binding my heart.

If I give myself altogether, the way
torenia gives its nectar

to the hummingbird, I'll lose you,
so I give it all to the sandwiches,

the avocado smoothed and spread
to hold sweet pickles to the sourdough.

I've never told you how your eyes
are the dazzle on the harbor.

I'm just the full moon, hesitating
in the daytime sky, cutting my losses.

FRED WANTS TO KNOW IF I BELIEVE IN GOD

At lunch, he asks me unironically.
A hush falls over our table—no context

here for such a question. I could say yes,
I do believe in a God I don't comprehend,

a wisp, or maybe a force stronger
than anything, far from me,

not a him or her, no robes, no arms, no legs.
I could say no to Fred, I don't believe

in your God. He's too small, too human.
And how could you still believe anyway,

Fred, after He took your daughter, gave her
a stupid infection from a fall in the road?

I feel a power near me or in me.
It grabs me when consciousness

leaks out of me, grabs
and shakes me alive.

TEMPORARY SEPARATION

I'm inside this body that doesn't work
the way it did before, as if all my angles

were filed down. Fear of falling makes me
consider where I sit, where I step.

Love is pulling me up. Every day
the children call. A gift of sequined silk

and flowers from my brother. You drive me
everywhere, carry and lift. Nights are long,

streetlights shining in through the curtains,
in the drizzle, the neighborhood

turned nineteenth century romantic,
but the surgeon has separated us as though

I'm covered in Post Office labels:
Fragile, Special Handling. There's a big scar

on my chest, and I'm afraid you might
bang into me with your elbows and knees.

I serve dinner by candlelight,
hoping it's a temporary separation.

DIGNITY

Dignity was hugely bloated,
with tubes in her orifices,
unconscious, not even knowing
nurses and aides cleaned her.
Dignity grasped for tiny clues
of what might be the future,
Dignity, who had never worn
a stretched-out T-shirt, had never
stepped outside without eye-liner,
lay in bed for weeks, missed
her hair appointment, and her roots
were showing. One whole night
she called out and couldn't stop.
When Dignity awoke, and saw
her family standing around her,
she thought about saying something
profound, like Dignity can be pick-
pocketed in an instant, but instead
she said, *my mother made Jello in July.*

MY CONCERNS ARE VERY SMALL

Today my blood is still
coursing a skittery
two-step, and a fancy
slanted checkerboard floater
has moved into my eye,
zinging so fast I can't catch it.
Sometimes its slower sister
comes along, curvier, blowsier,
occluding my vision. In this time
of warning and powerlessness,
my concerns are picayune.
Tonight's super moon,
so unnaturally brilliant,
might have come from another
solar system to cast its rose-gold
over the harbor, its perigee
about to touch the water.

REBIRTH

Fall clean-up time came and went.
Tomato plants, scrambled in the raised bed,
laid down their lives for me.

Geraniums and vinca held on
until November. Still, rosemary stands,
an offering among dead chives.

The mess embarrasses me, but indoors
I forget about it, caught up in the work
of stretching my back, lifting small weights,

making chocolate-avocado pudding,
I carry my own bags, stuffed with a book
of psalms, Ta-Nehisi Coates' novel,

a spirometer to strengthen my lungs,
a manuscript of poems. As winter light
increases, I am lighter, my legs no longer

resisting forward motion. So strange
after the surgery, lumpy and inert, my body
is becoming familiar again, answering to me.

Come spring, I'll clear the garden,
fill the beds with seeds and flowers,
witness the blooming.

UNDER A GIANT HAT

If, as my 4-year-old granddaughter said,
the sky is a Giant Hat
and everyone is wearing it.
Does that include me?
Am I under the hat, trying
to convince myself I'm still here?

I'm more than the hours I toss at night,
more than the twinges
in my chest that scare me,

more than the things that encircle me:
the sea, my poems, my paintings,
my nights, more than
the surfaces to pierce with words.

I'm cooking, the sun at my back,
dried porcini giving off its musk,
      the dark broth, ephemeral.
           My step feels so light.

ODE TO YOUR BREATH

You filled your lungs and breathed yourself
into me until the ambulance came,

steady breath as you drove through
the night, called for our children.

Deep sighing breath when I screamed
your name and you knew I was alive.

Shallow breath the motionless weeks
you listened in case I needed you.

Caught-in-your-throat breath as you held me
upright in the shower, and while I walked

unsteady through unfamiliar streets,
your hand tight in mine.

You let out a sobbing breath for uncertainty,
for what you almost lost.

A DAY WE EAT LIKE GODS

making its small explosions on the water,
    a luminescent day brushed by dawn,

        fog obscuring the opposite shore, the town and the boats,

              as though the indefinite world were dissolving,

      a benign day, blue, a foreign blue, distant, hopeful—
            cerulean water bluer than cerulean sky,

        and all the blue varieties of clouds tumble over themselves,

  a ravenous day we eat like gods,
      bright acid of the garden's tomatoes,
          stone fruits—their sweetness decomposing in the dish,
      elderberries ripening to be pressed into cordial,
        vine leaves, rolled around rice,

  a day pouring slow and predictable as if through capillaries.

AFTER MY YEAR OF BEING TWO-DIMENSIONAL

Nothing to say we haven't said before,
one year after my aorta burst.
Nothing to do to mark this date you call
my birthday, the anniversary of my luck,
the planets aligning, the helpers knowing
exactly how to grab me from the clutch.
No tunnel of light, only the nothing
that lurked just at the edge. You sit
on the bed and we look at each other long.
My brother calls to say *one year later
and better than ever*—my survival registering
to a tiny circle in a world spinning
out of control. I'll shower after my
twenty-two minutes with Jane Fonda whose
plastic surgeon must be phenomenal.
I wouldn't do it—too afraid of being
immutably unrecognizable. In the blaze
of today, we go in the ocean, silky,
billowing toward a horizon smudged
like the future. Ice cream for dessert,
a spectacular sunset, a few dark blue clouds.
Now you cry over the kitchen sink.
I end the day writing a thank you
to the doctor who saved my life,
a former journalist who changed
his career after Chechnya.

ABOUT THEIR VIGIL

They kept touching each other,
that touch a small solace, a begging:
stay, please. Don't stop breathing,
the whole week I was comatose,
time ticking away between their palms.

They weren't tired or hungry, didn't
notice rain or heat or twilight in this
narrow hopescape. Sadness, too,
could begin later. Nothing now
but the waiting, the days cresting
with messages from the doctors.

When the rabbi came, they spoke to her,
grasping at her connection
to holy power. At night, they'd
phone each other from bed
in their separate rooms.

When they knew I would live,
they wondered. How? Vegetative?
Or would I still dig quahogs,
paint storm clouds and elephants?

When I woke, I said the commotion
in my throat was nuclear. *Normal*,
they said, and held each other in relief.

NOTHING IS THE SAME

On the deck of the cabin
under the Perseids, my children
slept close to their father,
stars falling all around them.
I stayed inside, afraid of small
wild animals sniffing my face.
And weren't they also together after
my heart surgery, seeing me bloated,
distorted? They didn't believe
I'd come out whole to bake granola bars,
color my hair. An outline of myself I was,
a minute by minute report on the screen.
Weeks I don't remember—
shower, go to sleep, climb stairs.
Up, insurmountable. Down, a slip
off a precipice. Now, my son wants to know
what I'm cooking every day. My daughter
needs to know that I am.
I'm back, I want to shout.
Isn't this enough?

A MEDITATION ON THE PRESENT

The peas I planted too late,
the sharp bite of them, I pick,
sauté, butter and feed you,
the anniversary
of my near-death upon us.
Should we celebrate?
I don't know how, except
to keep breathing.
The fawn has come into the yard
again, her observant ears
big and tense, the rest of her so thin,
she's almost two-dimensional.
I stare and she stares back at me.
The few lilies she has
left after eating, shout out
yellow, emphatic and clear,
like the shirts of the mothers standing
arm-in-arm against injustice.
As alizarin crimson streaks
across the darkening sky,
the elderberries are ripening,
into bluish-black fruit
I'll turn into cordial,
the ripening missed last year
when I almost was recovering.
I will float on any small disturbance
that can rock me
from my impotence.

TONIGHT ONLY POETRY WILL SERVE

after Adrienne Rich

Only poetry will fly among the planets,
the stars, the new moon,
and my unconscious.
Awakened from coma,
there's a Chernobyl in my throat, I said,
a metaphor on my tongue.

Only poetry will stand me up
on a scallop shell naked in my wavy hair
while the nurses shower me, scrub my back,
and I hold on, grateful to be upright,
oblivious to everyone elsewhere,
standing or not.

And only poetry will pull me
word by word by word
to the table where I write
verb, noun, participle,
sometimes a reckless adjective.
I am returned.

ACKNOWLEDGMENTS

Many thanks to the following journals who gave these poems their first homes:

Bellevue Literary Review: "Temporary Separation," forthcoming.
River Styx: "I Must Have Been Wild for Life" and "Letting Go," 2021.
Ruminate: "Fred Wants to Know if I Believe in God," 2021.

I am everlastingly grateful to my husband, David, for knowing what to do, and to the others who saved my life—the Mattapoisett Police EMTs, Dr. Matthew Bivens and the staff at St. Luke's Emergency Department in New Bedford, and to Dr. Venkatachalam Senthilnathan, my surgeon at Beth Israel Deaconess Medical Center.

Thank you to the people at Spaulding Rehab, to my son, Ben, who calls me every day from Oregon, and to Sasha, my daughter, for her daily communication with that huge circle of the worried, to my brother, Peter, my extended family, friends and neighbors for their love, help, and rehab support.

Thank you to my writing community—which includes the group that began around my table, the members we added on Zoom, and the Mattapoisett poets—for editing the sentimentality out of these poems.

Thank you to Eileen Cleary for her validation and commitment to this book.

ABOUT THE AUTHOR

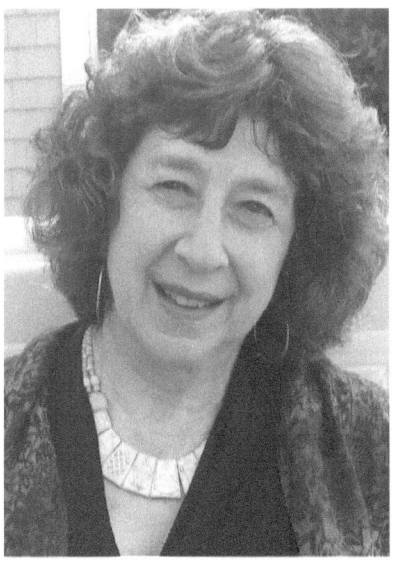

Margot Wizansky's poems have appeared online and in many journals such as *The American Journal of Poetry, Missouri Review, Bellevue Literary Review, Ruminate, River Styx, Cimarron*, and elsewhere. She edited two anthologies: *Mercy of Tides: Poems for a Beach House*, and *Rough Places Plain: Poems of the Mountains*. She won two residencies, one with Writers@Work in Salt Lake City and also with Carlow University in Sligo, Ireland. Margot is retired from a career developing housing for adults with disabilities. She lives in Massachusetts.

www.ingramcontent.com/pod-product-compliance
Lightning Source LLC
Chambersburg PA
CBHW020915080526
44589CB00011B/614